HEMORRHOIDS

DIFFERENT MEANS FOR HEALING PILES

DR. A. RAMOS

Contents

INTRODUCTION

Pain and bleeding are caused by hemorrhoids, commonly referred to as piles, which are enlarged and inflamed veins in the rectum and anus. Both internal and external vascular structures may be present, and elevated pressure in the lower rectum is frequently the root cause. A sedentary lifestyle, pregnancy, straining during bowel movements, and obesity are some of the factors that can lead to hemorrhoids, which are a common condition that affect people of all ages. Though they're usually not dangerous, hemorrhoids can cause discomfort, itching, and bleeding, which prompts people to look for relief through a variety of therapies and lifestyle changes.

CHAPTER ONE

The Meaning of Hemorrhoids

Vascular structures in the anal canal that enlarge and inflame are known as hemorrhoids, or piles. Blood vessels, muscle, and connective tissue make up these structures. The two locations of hemorrhoids are under the skin surrounding the anus on the outside and inside the rectum.

Eroded pelvic and rectal vein pressure is the main cause of hemorrhoids. Numerous factors, such as the following, may contribute to this pressure.

Breathing Through Straining: Hemorrhoids may develop as a result of prolonged breathing through straining during bowel movements.

The development of hemorrhoids can be attributed to conditions such as constipation or diarrhea that cause recurrent bowel movements or difficulty passing stools.

Pregnancy: Menstruating women are more likely to experience hemorrhoids due to hormonal fluctuations and the increased pressure on the pelvic area.

Fat: Being overweight raises the risk of hemorrhoids by putting pressure on the rectal veins.

Extended Sitting: Hemorrhoids can develop as a result of a sedentary lifestyle, which includes prolonged sitting.

An age-related increase in the risk of hemorrhoids is common.

Pain, itching, bleeding during bowel movements, and a lump near the anus are all possible signs of hemorrhoids. Hemorrhoids are thought to be a relatively benign medical condition, despite the fact that they can be uncomfortable. Aside from dietary and lifestyle modifications, topical creams and, in certain situations, medical procedures are available as forms of treatment. To ensure a precise diagnosis and suitable treatment of hemorrhoids, consulting a physician is essential.

Internal and external hemorrhoids are the two primary types of hemorrhoids that can be distinguished by location. The veins that are swollen and inflamed within the anal canal and surrounding the anus determine the classification.

Internal bleeding

Less pain is experienced by internal hemorrhoids because they form inside the rectum, which has fewer pain-sensing nerves. According to their severity, they are divided into four stages:

The first degree of hemorrhoids is characterized by bleeding without prolapse, or bleeding outside the anal opening.

In the second degree, bleeding occurs when the colon retracts and prolapses on its own.

Third Degree: The need for manual prolapse pushing back during bowel movements.

Fourth Grade: Prolapse that is unrepairable; they may have blood clots or pull a large portion of the rectum's lining through the anus.

Outer Hemorrhoids:

On the skin's outer edge surrounding the anal opening, external hemorrhoids form. During sitting or when having a bowel movement, they can cause pain or itching. They may also bleed when irritated. Blood clots in enlarged veins can cause severe pain and swelling, which is what happens to thrombosed external hemorrhoids.

When both internal and external hemorrhoids are present at the same time, it is possible for an individual to have a condition called mixed hemorrhoids.

The right treatment strategy must be chosen after taking into account the type and severity of hemorrhoids. If the condition is more severe, surgery or medical procedures may be necessary, but mild cases can often be treated with lifestyle modifications and over-the-counter medications. To effectively manage hemorrhoids, it is crucial to seek medical advice for an accurate diagnosis and customized treatment plan.

The reasons and elements that contribute

Vascular pressure in the rectal and anal regions is frequently elevated when hemorrhoids develop. Hemorrhoids can develop as a result of a variety of circumstances and actions.

Rigidity During Discharge:

The development of hemorrhoids can be facilitated by prolonged and vigorous straining during bowel movements, which can raise the pressure on the rectal veins.

Long-term diarrhea or constipation:

Haemorrhoids can develop in the rectal area as a result of conditions that cause persistent diarrhea or constipation. Anxiety may be made worse by irregular bowel movements.

A pregnancy

Pregnant women may be more vulnerable to hemorrhoids due to the altered hormone levels and increased pressure on the pelvic area.

The state of obesity

Obese people have a higher risk of hemorrhoids due to the increased pressure that excess body weight puts on the pelvic veins.

Spending Extended Times Sitting:

Hemorrhoids can develop as a result of a sedentary lifestyle, particularly when sitting still for long periods of time. In the rectal region, immobility impairs blood circulation.

Old

With age comes an increased risk of hemorrhoids. The anal and rectal connective tissues may deteriorate with age in people.

DNA Propensity:

Hemorrhoids may run in families, making a person more prone to the ailment.

Large-scale lifting:

Hemorrhoids can develop as a result of elevated intra-abdominal pressure, which can be caused by heavy lifting or straining while lifting weights.

Long-term Sneezing or Coughing

Anxiety-producing illnesses that produce frequent coughing or sneezing can raise abdominal and rectal pressure, which may result in hemorrhoids.

Sexual Relations Anal:

Anaerobic sex can irritate and put more strain on the rectal veins, which can lead to the development of hemorrhoids.

Low Consumption of Fiber:

Hemorrhoids and straining during bowel movements can result from a low-fiber diet. Constipation can also cause other health problems.

Bowel Diseases with Inflammation (IBD):

Crohn's disease and ulcerative colitis are examples of chronic inflammatory diseases that can raise the risk of hemorrhoids develop.

To reduce the risk of hemorrhoids, people can adopt preventive measures and lifestyle modifications by being aware of these causes and contributing factors. Colorectal health can be improved by leading a healthy lifestyle that includes eating a diet high in fiber, drinking plenty of water, and getting regular exercise.

The signs and symptoms

Different types and degrees of hemorrhoids can cause different symptoms, and the severity of these symptoms can also vary. The following are typical signs of hemorrhoids:

Bleeding in the rectum:

One of the most typical signs of hemorrhoids is bleeding when passing gas. On toilet paper, in the toilet bowl, or on the surface of stools, bright red blood may be observed.

Anguish or Unease:

Another typical symptom that is frequently experienced is pain or discomfort around the anal area, particularly during and following bowel movements. More obvious pain, especially when sitting, may be experienced from external hemorrhoids.

Asthma and Skin Rashes:

Due to the presence of swollen and inflamed veins, itching and irritation can happen in the anal region.

Anus-Related Swelling or Lump:

A visible swelling or lump near the anal opening may be the result of external hemorrhoids. During self-examination, one can sense or see this.

Bowel Movement Protrusion:

A person may need to manually push internal hemorrhoids back into the anal opening if they prolapse or protrude outside during bowel movements.

Mucosal Discharge:

A mucous discharge that can irritate the wound even more is experienced by some people who have internal hemorrhoids.

Sensation of Partial Detoxification:

Patients suffering from hemorrhoids might feel as though their bowel movements are not entirely empty.

Blood Clot/Thrombosis:

An hard lump near the anus and excruciating pain can be symptoms of thrombosed external hemorrhoids, which are caused by blood clots forming within enlarged veins.

Notably, these symptoms can also be indicative of other rectal and anal conditions, even though they are characteristic of hemorrhoids. Patients should see a doctor for a proper diagnosis and appropriate treatment if they have severe or persistent symptoms. Exams can be performed by medical professionals, especially gastroenterologists or colorectal specialists, to identify the underlying cause of symptoms and suggest appropriate treatments.

Medical Evaluation and Diagnosis

Medical evaluations performed by healthcare providers are usually necessary to diagnose hemorrhoids. This is a possible sequence of events:

CHAPTER TWO

Medical Background:

The medical history of the patient, including the onset and course of symptoms, will be enquired about by the healthcare provider. Additionally, lifestyle factors, dietary habits, and bowel habits may be considered as potential risk factors for hemorrhoids.

Examining the body:

The rectal and anal regions are frequently examined physically. An external hemorrhoid may be visually inspected by the healthcare provider, and other abnormalities such as internal hemorrhoids or rectal bleeding may be evaluated by using a gloved, lubricated finger.

Rectal Examined Digitally (DRE)

An oiled, gloved finger is inserted into the rectum by the medical professional performing a digital rectal examination in order to feel for anomalies, such as internal hemorrhoids.

Analyzing the Anus Visually

An examination of the anal region visually can frequently be used to diagnose external hemorrhoids. Inflammation, swelling, and other outward symptoms may be observed by the medical professional.

Anascopy versus proctoscopy:

A lit tube is used to more thoroughly inspect the rectum and anal canal during a proctoscopy or anoscopy. As a result, the internal hemorrhoids can be thoroughly inspected.

A sigmoidoscopy or a colonoscopy

Occasionally, a sigmoidoscopy or colonoscopy may be advised, particularly if there are concerns regarding additional possible colorectal problems. For the purpose of visualizing the entire lower gastrointestinal tract, a flexible tube equipped with a camera is inserted into the colon or rectum.

Imaging Studies:

Under certain circumstances, imaging studies to obtain more details about the gastrointestinal tract like a barium enema or other radiographic imaging may be ordered.

If someone is bleeding, hurting, or uncomfortable, it's critical that they see a doctor for a proper diagnosis if they have hemorrhoids. Due to the possibility of hemorrhoids sharing symptoms with other colorectal conditions, a complete medical evaluation is necessary for an accurate diagnosis and the best course of treatment. After a diagnosis, depending on the type and severity of hemorrhoids, medical professionals may suggest topical treatments, lifestyle changes, or more involved interventions.

Depending on the severity and kind of the hemorrhoids, treatment usually consists of a mix of lifestyle changes, household remedies, and medical interventions. Here are some different treatment modalities:

Changing one's diet and lifestyle:

High-Fiber Diet: Eating a high-fiber diet reduces the pressure on the rectal veins by softening stools and encouraging regular bowel movements.

Getting enough water in your diet is important for maintaining intestinal health and preventing constipation.

Exercise on a regular basis: Frequent exercise helps to improve pelvic circulation and encourage regular bowel movements.

External Therapies:

Hydrocortisone is one ingredient that may be present in over-the-counter (OTC) creams and ointments to reduce inflammation and itching. But rather than being a permanent fix, they are mainly for symptom relief.

Spa Baths (Warm Baths):

For pain and discomfort relief, sitz baths, which involve soaking the anal area in warm water for 15 to 20 minutes, can help. Several times a day, this can be accomplished.

Topical Anaesthetics and Pelvic Administers:

Sponges can be used to administer medication by inserting them into the rectum, and topical anesthetics can be used to temporarily numb the area.

Rubber Band Ligation, also known as hemorrhoid banding,

In order to stop an internal hemorrhoid's blood supply, a rubber band is wrapped around its base during this procedure. At some point, during bowel movements, the hemorrhoid falls off.

IR Coagulation (IRC):

Hemorrhoid blood vessels are coagulated by infrared light used by IRC, which causes the hemorrhoid to contract.

Sclerotherapy

The hemorrhoid shrinks and eventually goes away when a chemical solution is injected into its blood vessels.

Hemorrhageectomy:

In extreme situations or after all other treatments have failed, surgical excision of hemorrhoids may be considered. For external hemorrhoids, it occurs more frequently.

Stapled hemorrhoidopexy, also known as hemorrhoid packing:

The hemorrhoid will shrink as a result of the procedure's use of staples to stop blood flow.

Excision of the throat:

An expert in healthcare may remove the blood clot and relieve pain and swelling in hemorrhoids that are thrombosed external (blood clot-ridden).

Getting a proper diagnosis and figuring out the best course of action based on unique circumstances require speaking with a healthcare professional. More sophisticated treatments might be necessary for severe or chronic hemorrhoids, while home cures and lifestyle modifications might be helpful for mild cases.

Prevention Techniques

The chance of getting hemorrhoids or stopping them from reoccurring can be significantly reduced by taking preventive action. In order to help avoid hemorrhoids, consider the following tactics:

Uphold a Diet Rich in Fiber:

Incorporate a diet rich in whole grains, legumes, fruits, and vegetables. Straining during defecation is less likely when fiber aids soften stools and encourages regular bowel motions.

Continue to drink water:

To avoid constipation and preserve ideal intestinal health, make sure you are drinking enough water throughout the day.

Regular Exercise:

Constipation can be avoided and general health can be enhanced by frequent exercise. Improved intestinal regularity can be attained through exercises like swimming, running, or walking.

Keep Your Bowel Movements Unrestrained:

Refrain from straining and take your time when passing the stool. To improve comfort during the procedure, utilize a stool softener if necessary.

Develop Good Toilet Practices:

Recess pressure on the area around the rectal valve can be increased by extended sitting on the toilet. To get a more natural position for bowel movements, you might also think about elevating your feet using a little step bench.

Sustain a Balanced Weight:

With a balanced diet and frequent exercise, you can reach and stay at a healthy weight. Recessive vein pressure might be exacerbated by being overweight.

Don't Stand or Sit for Long:

Take pauses to increase blood circulation and walk around if your profession needs you to sit or stand for extended periods of time.

Wear Loose-Fitting Clothing:

Choose loose-fitting, comfortable clothing to reduce unwanted pressure on the anal and rectal areas.

Practice Good Anal Hygiene:

Gently clean the anal area after bowel movements with mild, unscented wipes or moistened toilet paper. Avoid vigorous rubbing, which might irritate the skin.

Address Diarrhea or Constipation Promptly:

If you experience chronic diarrhea or constipation, get medical counsel to address the underlying causes and prevent strain on the rectal veins.

Incorporate Fiber Supplements:

If it's tough to get enough fiber from your diet, consider fiber supplements after talking with a healthcare expert.

Regular Health Check-ups:

Schedule regular check-ups with a healthcare practitioner to monitor and manage any underlying issues that may contribute to the development of hemorrhoids.

By following these preventive steps, individuals can dramatically minimize the risk of developing hemorrhoids and increase overall colorectal health. If symptoms or concerns occur, it's crucial to seek medical counsel for proper diagnosis and direction on suitable interventions.

Lifestyle Adjustments

Lifestyle modifications can contribute to the management and prevention of hemorrhoids. Here are some lifestyle adjustments that may help ease symptoms and lessen the risk of developing hemorrhoids:

High-Fiber Diet:

Include lots of fiber-rich items in your diet, such as fruits, vegetables, whole grains, and legumes. Fiber softens feces and facilitates regular bowel movements, lowering the strain on the rectal veins.

Adequate Hydration:

Drink enough water throughout the day to maintain hydration and support good bowel function. Hydration helps avoid constipation, a common component in hemorrhoid formation.

CHAPTER THREE

Regular Exercise:

Engage in frequent physical activity to increase overall health and improve bowel regularity. Activities like walking, jogging, or swimming can be useful.

Avoid Prolonged Sitting:

Take breaks from prolonged sitting, especially if you have a sedentary work. Stand, stretch, and move around occasionally to promote blood circulation in the rectal area.

Proper Toilet Habits:

Take your time during bowel movements, and avoid straining. Use a stool softener if needed to make bowel motions more comfortable. To get a more natural position for bowel movements, you might also think about elevating your feet using a little step bench.

Sustain a Balanced Weight:

With a balanced diet and frequent exercise, you can reach and stay at a healthy weight. Recessive vein pressure might be exacerbated by being overweight.

Wear Loose-Fitting Clothing:

Choose loose-fitting, comfortable clothing to reduce unwanted pressure on the anal and rectal areas.

Good Anal Hygiene:

Gently clean the anal area after bowel movements with mild, unscented wipes or moistened toilet paper. Avoid vigorous rubbing, which might irritate the skin.

Spa Baths (Warm Baths):

Soak the anal area in warm water for 15-20 minutes, known as sitz baths, to ease pain and discomfort. Several times a day, this can be accomplished.

Avoid Irritants:

Avoid using harsh soaps or perfumed items in the anal area, since these might cause inflammation.

Kegel Exercises:

Kegel exercises, which strengthen the pelvic floor muscles, may aid improve blood circulation in the rectal area and minimize the incidence of hemorrhoids.

Regular Health Check-ups:

Schedule regular check-ups with a healthcare practitioner to assess overall health and treat any concerns related to hemorrhoids.

These lifestyle improvements can help to better colon health and may give relief for persons having hemorrhoid discomfort. It's crucial to consult with a healthcare expert for specific guidance and to address any persistent or severe symptoms.

CONCLUSION

In conclusion, hemorrhoids are a common and frequently controllable ailment that involves the swelling and inflammation of veins in the rectum and anus. While they can cause discomfort, pain, and bleeding, implementing specific lifestyle changes and treatment measures can effectively ease symptoms and avoid their recurrence.

Key items to consider:

Prevention through Lifestyle:

Lifestyle modifications, such as maintaining a high-fiber diet, staying hydrated, engaging in regular exercise, and adopting correct toilet habits, play a key role in preventing hemorrhoids.

Symptom Management:

For individuals experiencing symptoms like bleeding, pain, or discomfort, numerous at-home therapies, including warm baths, topical treatments, and dietary adjustments, can provide relief.

Medical Interventions:

Medical therapies range from over-the-counter lotions and suppositories to more complex procedures like banding, infrared coagulation, and surgical options for severe instances.

Regular Health Check-ups:

Regular health check-ups with a healthcare professional are vital for monitoring general colorectal health, addressing issues, and discussing preventive actions.

Personalized Treatment Plans:

Treatment plans for hemorrhoids should be individualized based on the degree, kind, and individual circumstances. Consultation with a healthcare expert helps select the most relevant interventions.

By implementing preventive measures, making lifestyle adjustments, and obtaining prompt medical guidance when needed, individuals can effectively manage hemorrhoids and enhance their overall colorectal well-being. Hemorrhoids, while a common occurrence, can be managed with a combination of self-care, medical interventions, and a proactive approach to colorectal health.

THE END